INTERMITTENT FASTING

6 effective methods to lose weight, build muscle, increase your metabolism, get ketogenic, and get healthy

Table of Contents

Free Bonuses

As Promised Here Is Your FREE Cheat Sheet to Fat-Adapted Diets That I Use With My Clients

Go Here To Get Your Copy
http://eostre.us/index.php/ebooks-2/

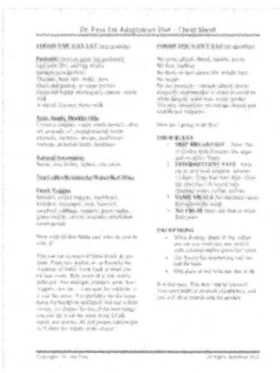

If You Want Free Best Selling Kindle Books Delivered to Your Inbox On A Weekly Basis

http://eostre.us/index.php/ebooks/

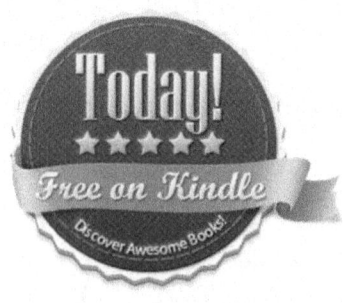

About the Author

Dr. Dan Foss graduated from Western States Chiropractic College in 2003. His fresh outlook on health, nutrition, and exercise has helped thousands of people not only get well but stay well for a lifetime. His goal as a Chiropractor is to help educate and empower people to understand how the human body works so that they can make the best decisions regarding their health and well-being. Over the last 13 years, he has practiced Chiropractic, and the last seven years has owned and operated Pura Vida Chiropractic, a wellness center based in San Antonio, Texas. When not practicing, he is a father, husband, coach, mentor, and amateur endurance athlete.

Other Books By This Author

I hope you enjoy reading this book! I have put a lot of work into studying and researching Intermittent Fasting, Ketogenic Diets, Low Carb High Fat Lifestyles, Fat Adaptation, and Heart Rate Training.

I have some other books on Amazon, and you might find something interesting or useful in them. Below is a list of my other books, along with direct links to their web-pages.

Ketogenic Diet Plan: 30 Day Meal Plan, 50 Ketogenic Fat Burning Recipes for Rapid Weight Loss and Unstoppable Energy

Low Carb High Fat 101: 20+ Best Recipes and Weekly LCHF Meal Plan, LCHF Explained, Ketogenic Diet and Fat Adapted Training.

Medical Disclaimer

My patients have benefited from the practice and even from the mere knowledge of methods of intermittent fasting and how the human body in general handles fat as an energy source, bountiful energy that is available both for the body's internal functions (including mental functions), and for any activities the person is involved in. But <u>there are nevertheless certain groups of people who in their current physical condition should not attempt intermittent fasting, or any fasting for that matter</u>. A list of medical or natural conditions people might be undergoing or afflicted by, which could make fasting an uncomfortable or even a risky experience in terms of their health is discussed in Chapter 8 of this book. You, the reader is cautioned to exercise wisdom if you are not relatively healthy, especially in combining fasting with strenuous physical exercise, and to consult with your personal doctor or physician before attempting any of the described methods of fasting in this book. Still, wisely followed, generally, methods of intermittent fasting can help most people attain better health, since the fasted body is permitted to rectify itself biologically on its own, to the degree it can.

You understand that any information as found within this book is for general educational and informational purposes only. You understand that such information is not intended nor otherwise implied to be medical advice.

You understand that such information is by no means complete or exhaustive, and that <u>as a result</u>, such information does not encompass all conditions, disorders, health-related issues, or respective treatments. You understand that you should always consult your physician or other healthcare provider to determine the appropriateness of this information for your own situation or should you have any questions regarding a medical condition or treatment plan.

You understand that the products and any related claims for such products might not been evaluated by the United States Food and Drug Administration (USFDA) and might not have been approved to diagnose, treat, cure or prevent disease. As such, you acknowledge that you are not relying in any fashion that the USFDA has approved such products and claims.

You agree not to use any information in this book, including, but not limited to product descriptions, customer testimonials, etc. for the diagnosis and treatment of any health issue or for the prescription of any medication or treatment.

You acknowledge that all testimonials as found in our book are strictly the opinion of that person, and any results such person may have achieved are solely individual in nature; your results may vary.

You understand that such information is based upon personal experience and is not a substitute for obtaining professional medical advice. You should always consult your physician or other healthcare provider before changing your diet or starting an exercise program.

In light of the forgoing, you understand and agree that we are not liable nor do we assume any liability for any information contained within this book as well as your reliance on it. In no event shall we be liable for direct, indirect, consequential, special, exemplary, or other damages related to your use of the information contained within our book.

This book offers health, fitness and nutritional information and is designed for informational and educational purposes only. You should not rely on this information as a substitute for professional medical advice, nor does it replace professional medical advice, diagnosis, or treatment. Please discuss all your medical and nutritional questions with your health-care provider. If you have any concerns or questions about your health, you should always consult with a physician or other health-care professional.

The Food and Drug Administration have not evaluated the statements made within this book. The statements mentioned in this book are not intended to diagnose, treat, cure or prevent any disease.

Do not disregard, avoid or delay obtaining medical or health-related advice from your health-care professional because of something you may have read in this book. The use of any information provided in this book is solely at your own risk.

Developments in medical research may impact the accuracy of health, fitness and nutritional information that appears in this book. No assurance can be given that the information contained in this book will always include the most recent findings or developments with respect to the particular material.

The information provided by this book is believed to be accurate at the time it was created and it was based on research and on our best judgment. However, like any

Introduction

Thank you for taking the time to download this book: "Intermittent Fasting: 6 effective methods to lose weight, build muscle, increase your metabolism, get *ketogenic*, and get healthy."

This book covers the topic of intermittent fasting, and will teach you what it is, different ways it is done, and why it may be a good idea for you to try it. The book goes over several different routines and schedules you can chose from. The important thing to know about intermittent fasting is that it is not a diet but instead a window of time in which to eat your calories. You will not necessarily eat more or fewer calories than you are eating now.

Human beings have not always eaten every 3-4 hours like we tend to do today, and our bodies are designed to survive and even thrive without eating so frequently. Just like in the Paleolithic era our cavemen and cave-women ancestors had to hunt and kill their food, so our bodies are accustomed to hunting and gathering our food and storing it for the winter or tough times. You might be surprised at how easily your body can adjust to adding fasting periods to your daily life. The modern human being eats not only more than ever but also more frequently than ever.

One of the most wonderful things about intermittent fasting is that it is so simple, you are likely to stick to it; and it is powerful enough that you should quickly see results! Also, fasting is a completely cost-free way of changing your life and losing weight, so you can start today! In reality, fasting will probably save you money! It is also more flexible than many other weight-loss diets, allowing you to tailor it to your specific lifestyle.

How do you know what method is right for you? Be realistic about your personality, your level of willpower, and your lifestyle. Can you handle not having a huge breakfast on Sundays? Can you see yourself not eating for a full 24 hours? These are the questions you can only answer for yourself.

At the completion of this book, you will have a good understanding of how to start an intermittent fast, what to eat while fasting, how to do physical training or exercise while fasting, what the health benefits are, and some science behind it all.

Once again, thanks for downloading this book, I hope you find it to be helpful!

Chapter 1: Overview of Intermittent Fasting

Intermittent fasting is gaining popularity as a method to lose weight and feel healthier. Fasting is something that has long been done by humans, either because food was not readily available, or for religious reasons. Many people consider periods of fasting to be more natural than eating 3-4 meals per day, every day. The human body is designed to function without eating for much greater periods of time.

The main concept of intermittent fasting is combining periods of not eating with periods of eating. There are several different ways this is accomplished, six of which I'll discuss in the next chapter.

It has been suggested that intermittent fasting may be more effective for men than women. But in studies on both have seen positive results. Yet, people prone to eating disorders should probably not try fasting without first finding an alternative method of dieting.

Most people would be initially concerned about how they will feel when they start intermittent fasting. You may worry that you will be a grouch in the morning if you skip your breakfast, for instance. The truth is: you might be, at least at first. The idea that people have to eat every 3 hours or so is a mental thing. You may have to retrain your mind so it understands the body does not need food so often to survive.

Think about fasting as a method of cleansing your body. Your body scavenges your body for free radicals and damaged cells during these periods and recycles them to conserve energy.

Why are people turning to intermittent fasting more and more? Here is a list of some of the many benefits:

- <u>You lose weight</u>. Intermittent fasting can help you lose weight, specifically, belly fat, and with some of these methods of fasting you do not have to restrict your calorie intake. Short-term fasting can also increase your metabolism rate, so it is helping on both sides of the calorie equation which determines fat buildup (calories-in vs. calories-out). Go here for reference **http://eostre.us/ifmetab**

- <u>It may slow down aging</u>. Studies involving lab rats showed that rats that fasted on and off lived 36-83% longer than those who were given rations of food daily. Go here for reference **https://www.scientific american.com/article/how-intermittent-fasting-might-help-you-live-longer-healthier-life/**

- <u>It's good for your brain</u>. Intermittent fasting has been shown to increase the production of the brain hormone BDNF (*Brain-derived neurotrophic factor*), which may help grow new nerve cells. Studies have also shown it may protect against Alzheimer's Disease. A 2007 study in the Journal of Neurobiology of Disease found mice with Alzheimer's Disease undergoing intermittent fasting performed better on memory tests compared to the control group with Alzheimer's Disease that was not put on intermittent fasting. Go here for Reference https://www.ncbi.nlm.nih.gov/pubmed/17306982

- It can add mental clarity to your life. Fat is technically one of the most fuel-efficient sources for your body to run on. Your brain consumes a huge portion of the energy you use. Training your body to run on fat reserves can help reduce mental fogginess and add mental clarity. This is called "fat adaptation" or "keto-adaptation". When you think of it, most of us have on average 40,000 calories of fat in our body (around our organs), compared to 1,200 to 1,500 calories of glycogen. Go here for Reference https://www.ncbi.nlm.nih.gov/pmc/articles/PMC36 70843/

- It lowers blood sugar. By fasting intermittently, your body lessens its insulin resistance. This can help prevent the development of type 2 Diabetes Mellitus. Go here for Reference https://www.ncbi.nlm.nih.gov /pmc/articles/PMC3670843/

- It's good for your heart. Some common lab test results point to the possibility of problems with the heart. They are: LDL cholesterol, inflammatory markers, blood triglycerides, and blood sugar. Intermittent fasting may help to reduce all of those levels and medical markers. In fact, new research on LDL's has shown that your LDL levels can be read two ways, not just as how much concentration you have in your blood: One is LDL-C or measure of the concentration; and the other is LDL-P or particle size of the LDL's. The larger particle size of LDL's indicates less of a health risk than an increase in LDL concentration. In other words: the smaller LDL particles suspended in your blood, are more directly associated with higher risk of heart problems, and not so much the quantity of LDL you may have in your blood. Alternate day fasting has been shown to increase LDL particle size independently of dietary fat content in obese people. Go here for Refernece https://www.ncbi.nlm.nih.gov/pubmed/23612508

- It may help prevent cancer. Several studies done on animals have suggested that intermittent fasting could possibly help prevent cancer. The intermittent-fasting calorie restriction has been correlated with a decreased IGF-1, a hormone linked to aging and cancer. Go here for Reference https://www.ncbi.nlm.nih.gov/pmc/articles/PMC2815756/

- It reduces inflammation. Certain studies of Intermittent Fasting have shown reductions in medical markers for inflammation, which is a main contributor to many chronic illnesses. Go here for Reference https://www.ncbi.nlm.nih.gov/pubmed/17291990/

In addition to all of the health benefits listed, it also simplifies your life. Having to make fewer meals frees up time to do other things. You have fewer meals to prepare and fewer trips to the supermarket. It is a relief for many people.

So what exactly is going on in your body while you are fasting? Some of the key changes your body goes through are:

- Cell Repair: When you are fasting, your body initiates processes such as *autophagy*, which is when each cell digest or otherwise uses up old and dysfunctional proteins and dead tissue that has built up within each cell.

- Insulin Drop: The levels of insulin in your blood drop and insulin sensitivity of the cells in the body improve greatly during a fast, which is the opposite effect than is observed in people with Diabetes II. Lower levels of insulin allow stored body fat to become more accessible.

- Human Growth Hormone (HGH): The levels of HGH increase substantially during a fast. There are many health benefits associated with this, including an increased ability to lose weight and build muscle. Other benefits of high levels of the HGH:
  - Strengthens your bones
  - Promotes healthy hair and nail growth
  - Improves circulation
  - Protects organs from the decline that occurs with age
  - Reduces some signs and indications of aging.

- Burn Stored Fat: After you eat, your body will digest and use the food you have just consumed for energy within the next few hours, and will then store the leftovers as fat. Intermittent fasting means your body is forced to turn to stored fats in order to get energy. This is called "*ketosis*", and the ability of your body to access these fats is called "*fat adaptation*".

When you are fasting, you need to limit your intake to water and other liquids such as coffee, and tea, or branch chain amino acids. Many people consider it an acceptable cheat to add a little coconut or whole milk to their coffee but the reality is: milk and coconut are high in calories.

Before beginning an intermittent fasting schedule, it is important to look at your diet. You will not have success if the calories you are eating are the wrong type of calories. If your diet consists of mostly processed foods, intermittent fasting may not be for you. The things you <u>do</u> want to include in your diet are vegetable carbohydrates, healthy proteins, and healthy fats. Examples of healthy fats include coconut oil, eggs, avocados, raw nuts, and olive oil.

Chapter 2: Six Popular Ways to Fast Intermittently

In order to be successful, consistent, and regular while fasting intermittently, you need to find a method that can fit into your lifestyle. Here are 6 popular ways to go about it.

1. **16/8 Method:** This method is so popular that the next chapter of this book is dedicated to explaining how to get started with it. Basically, it entails not eating for 16 hours each day of your fast, and then having an 8-hour window in which you can eat 2 to 3 meals. During the fasting period, it is fine to drink water or beverages that are non-caloric like tea or coffee. Simply do not eat anything after dinner and by the time lunch rolls around the next day it will probably have been around 16 hours. If you are someone that naturally skips breakfast, you may find it easy to adopt this method, also known as the "Leangains protocol". Many health experts recommend that women change the regime slightly and eat after 14-15 hours because they tend to do better with a slightly shorter fast. In order for this to be an effective weight loss method, it is important that you eat healthy meals during your 8-hour non-fasting window and not a bunch of processed or refined foods. Many people find it easy to adjust to this method of intermittent fasting and it becomes effortless to them. Pros of this method are, among others: it saves money because you are eating fewer

meals; you do not have to count calories; and it burns fat. A difficulty with this method is that it is very strict about what you can and cannot eat. It is good for people who consider themselves gym addicts and endurance athletes. Martin Berkhan developed this method.

2. **Eat-Stop-Eat:** In order to pull this off, you do a complete 24-hour fast either once or twice a week. The best way to accomplish this is to go from the end of a meal to the same meal-time the following day. An example being if you finish dinner at 7 pm on a Saturday, you would not eat again until 7 pm on Sunday or whenever you eat dinner. You can also go from breakfast to breakfast or from lunch to lunch, whatever is more convenient for your lifestyle. Again, water and any other non-caloric beverages are fine. Eat normally during the periods of eating, but aim for healthy foods over junk. You may find it too hard to go 24 hours right away and need to build up over time, starting with 15-16 hours at first and working your way from there. This method takes a lot of self-discipline but it may be preferable if you want to eat normally most of the week and focus your fasting to just a day or two. Pros of this method include that it requires less willpower because you know that your fast is short. You can also somewhat eat what you want as long as it is in moderation. Brad Pilon is credited with creating this method of intermittent fasting.

3. **The 5:2 Method/Diet:** This method is very similar to Eat-Stop-Eat, but does not require you to fast for a full 24 hours. To do this method, eat normally 5 days

a week and restrict yourself to 500-600 calories per day twice a week. Some studies suggest women are supposed to aim for 500 calories and men for 600. This is usually broken up into two small meals for the day. The two low-calorie counting days in which you somewhat fast should not be consecutive. This method has had the least amount of research done and critics are quick to point out that there are no scientific studies showing its effectiveness, therefore I cannot recommend it. Plus, this method does require you to keep track of the calories you are eating, so that's a disadvantage.

4. **The Warrior Method/Diet:** Fast all day, and then feast at night if you want to try this. This kind-of reminds me, and perhaps you too, of the Viking movies where the warriors come back to the lodge, and there are crates and plates of abundant foods awaiting. During the day, you are allowed to snack on fruits and vegetables as long as they are raw. Then, at night you eat one giant meal. You technically get a 4-hour window to eat at night, but most users of this method stick to one large meal. This method of fasting/dieting agrees with the *"Paleo"* diet in which people try to stick to healthy, natural, unprocessed foods that resemble what foods are found in Nature. Of all the diets to become popular in recent years, the warrior diet was the first to involve a type of intermittent fasting. Pros of this method are: 1) You can eat appropriate snacks, and 2) It is very, very healthy. The con is that you have to really monitor yourself and make sure you are making healthy food choices. Other than raw fruit and veggies, you are fasting for a full 20 hours every day. This method is

credited to Ori Hofmekler. There are some similarities to the Ramadan or the 30 day Muslim fast, with Ramadan of course being mostly spiritually motivated.

5. **Alternate Day Fasting:** If you are up to the challenge, you can try to fast every other day. This is an extreme method that should not be attempted by beginners, but you can choose to go with a full-on fast or to limit your calorie intake to about 500 every other day. Many of the scientific studies that showed health benefits of intermittent fasting used a sort of alternate day fasting. Ideally, while using this method, you are still eating at least once a day, with your fast going from dinnertime to dinnertime every other day. The pros of this type of fasting are: 1) you will experience rapid weight loss- with people averaging a 1 to 2 lbs. drop per week. 2) It requires less will power, for you eat a little on fasting days and you can look forward to eating more the next day. The con is that you have to be very, very careful to not binge on your eating days. Dr. James Johnson created this type of intermittent fasting when he realized it is clearly impossible for most working people to maintain a consistent calorie restriction by pure will power.

6. **Meal Skipping:** You do not need to follow an incredibly strict schedule to get some benefits from intermittent fasting. Today's market-oriented forces have convinced the majority that we need to eat every few hours or we will start losing muscle tone and begin to starve. If you are not feeling hungry or are too busy to stop and eat, simply skip a meal. Just

that, actually has some benefits. Generally speaking, and discomfort aside, the human body is configured in advance to handle up to a famine, so skipping a meal or two will not cause you any damage. Skipping a meal or two when it works out best for you is basically a spontaneous intermittent fast done in a very natural way. Just make sure that when you are eating, it is healthy food.

No matter what method of intermittent fasting you chose, it is important to reiterate the following: Remember to make good choices when picking your foods. It will not matter how long you fasted if you are gorging yourself on junk food during your eating periods.

There's another far less common method of intermittent fasting known as the "fast/feast" model, but I do not recommend it. In this regime, you eat whatever you want for a full 24 hours and then you fast for a full 36-hours. You then repeat the cycle for some time. It has been known to promote rapid weight loss. However, most people do not want to fast for that long, and they tend to "cheat" to such an extreme that the fast is therefore ineffective.

Chapter 3: The "16/8" Method Step-by-Step

The key is to exercise fasted, keeping your body in a Ketogenic state, so you are burning more fat for fuel than sugars.

No matter what type of diet you are trying, losing weight is a matter of "calories in" versus "calories out". (To lose weight, you must ingest less calories than your body used for all of its functions during a given time window.) The interesting thing about eating in an 8-hour window is: there is only so much that you can eat before you feel full. This means it is important to eat according to your expected energy expenditure and activity levels. Below, is an example of a menu you can use to start out the 16/8 Intermittent Fast.

My best recommendation's for your eating window of 8 hours depends on your exercise training schedule, or on your regular schedule if you don't exercise routinely. Typically, I recommend that you fast from 8pm, to 12pm of the next day. This gives you between 12pm to 8pm to eat. During your fasting time I recommend you consume only liquids and natural plant-based sweeteners.

From an exercise standpoint try to fast through the time when you normally exercise. While you fast, you can exercise in the morning right when you wake up, or just before lunchtime. The key is to exercise fasted keeping your body in a Ketogenic state so you are burning fat for fuel rather than sugars or simple carbohydrates.

Here is an example of a Ketonic diet plan for this method of fasting:

Day 1

Wake-Up time: You can have coffee, tea (non-caloric, without sugar), or water, whichever you choose

Morning: Again, stick to liquids like water, coffee, and tea and zero-calorie natural sweeteners like Stevia or Xylitol.

Lunch: Chicken breast with lots of leafy green vegetables or another protein source like meat, pork, fish, or turkey. Try to add some good fats like coconut or avocado.

Snacks: Nuts and Seeds are great snacks during the day.

Dinner: Have a dinner between 6 to 8 PM. Salmon (or another healthy fish or protein source) with vegetables.

Bedtime: Try to stop eating two hours before you go to sleep.

Day 2

Wake-Up: Same as day one, coffee or tea (non-caloric) to get you moving as needed.

Morning: Stick to the same liquids as day 1. Again go for natural sweeteners, not artificial ones.

Lunch: Protein with vegetables.

Snacks: Nuts, Seeds, or Berries

Dinner: Same two-hour window for eating one or two small meals. Try baked chicken breast with oven-roasted vegetables.

Bedtime: Always try to wait two hours after you eat to go to sleep.

Your diet will want to contain mainly unprocessed foods. Meat, fish, eggs, vegetables, and just a small amount of low glycemic fruit, is what your meals should consist of mostly. Processed foods tend to be very high in calories while being very low in nutritional value. If you feel you need a "cheat day", try to save that for the weekends.

Drink lots and lots of water. Try to drink at least ½ an ounce per day for every pound of your body weight. (For instance, a 130 lb. person would drink about 2 quarts per day; and about 3 quarts for someone weighing 190 lbs.) This seems like a lot of water but the reality is this will help keep you full and hydrated. The average person, typically thinks they are feeling hungry, when actually they are just feeling thirsty. Drinking water will help suppress feelings of hunger. You can also chew sugar-free gum to give your mouth something to do (and producing saliva). Studies have shown that some gums have certain sweeteners that turn into calories in your stomach, so make sure you are sticking to the sugar-free variety.

Traditionally, most exercise trainers and coaches have recommended eating a big breakfast or 4 to 5 balanced meals throughout the day. The 16/8 method skips breakfast as an extension of the natural overnight fast.

It is a good idea to use your fasting time to be productive. Sitting around and feeling hungry will only make things harder on yourself moving forward.

The 16/8 method is often used in combination with a strict exercise regime and as such should be used in combination with branch chain amino acids. How and when to use them will be discussed in the next chapter.

Also, if you are coupling your 16/8 intermittent fasting with an intense workout regime, it is recommended that you add more protein to your evening meal. Look for animal or plant based proteins, or a protein supplement.

Chapter 4: Supplementing the "16/8" with BCAAs

BCAA stands for branched chain amino acids, and if you are looking to gain muscle with intermittent fasting it is important for you to understand "amino acids" - what our bodies form proteins and muscle fiber out of. If your workout time falls during your fasting time, BCAAs allow you to work out, to lose fat without losing muscle.

There are three amino acids that are typically being referred to when people say BCAAs. Those are Valine, Leucine, and Isoleucine. (A common use of this type of supplementation is for people with low dietary protein intake.) BCAAs are also used to protect novice athletes from fatigue. When you are fasting, your body is not getting the flow of calories it is accustomed to. At that point BCAAs can help you stop the sense of fatigue.

Here is for instance how to use BCAAs to get the most out of your fasting and workout:

6:45 am:	10g (grams) of BCAAs
7:00 am:	Weight Training
9:00 am:	10g of BCAAs
11:00 am:	10g of BCAAs
1:00 pm:	Meal
4:00 pm:	Snack (optional)
8:00 pm:	Meal

This method can be useful for anyone trying to lose weight, gain muscle, and gain strength. It will improve your overall body composition.

Some things to note when exercising with BCAAs and on the 16/8 method:

- The feeding window should be kept somewhat consistent, as your body will get used to eating at certain times. Maintaining a routine will make the whole thing easier on you.

- BCAAs come in tablets and in powder form. Generally, the tablets are cheaper but less convenient. The powder can be mixed in the water bottle you take along. Drink the first third 5-15 minutes before you begin your workout, and another third every other hour.

- BCAAs in powder form by themselves, taste horrible. Some of them are mixed with aspartame or other artificial sweeteners to make them more palatable. My advice is to stay away from those, simply mix the pure powder with Stevia; or take the capsules.

- There are vegan BCAAs as well, and those type of amino acids are gaining in popularity.

Chapter 5: Exercise and Intermittent Fasting

One common question people have when doing intermittent fasting is whether or not it is safe and healthy to exercise either aerobically or anaerobically while they are, say, "running on empty". reak out the Jackson Browne! But, if done correctly, the combination can actually help you burn lots your body's fat reserves quickly. Maintaining some sort of exercise routine is vital for your mental and physical health – that's a given. So, in fact, exercising and running in a fasted state is a great way to become fat adapted and improve your mental state at the same time.

You've already heard the adage, 80% diet, 20% exercise – to combine dieting with exercise. This is true! Imagine if we could make our body burn more fat for fuel while at rest, and then also burn fat more efficiently during exercise. Like I mentioned in a previous chapter most of us have 40,000 calories of fat in our bodies at any given time, and around 1,200 calories of muscle glycogen or sugar. Imagine how far or how much we could exercise if we had access to that 40,000-calorie fuel tank. That's 33 times the amount of energy fuel! So, perhaps next time you run out of energy in the middle of an exercise routine, you will wish your body was in fat-burning mode instead of calorie-burning mode.

The first step to burning more fat during exercise is: you need to have what's called an "aerobic base." The way to build this base is thru aerobic heart rate training, which will raise what is known as your "aerobic capacity". Aerobic capacity is defined as the maximal amount of oxygen in milliliters (ml) that an athlete utilizes in one minute, per kilogram of body weight. In layman's terms, the higher the "aerobic base" or "capacity", the more body-work you can do in one minute. The best method I have found for heart rate training is Phil Maffetone's "MAF" training. I have included a link to his paper on heart rate training here, https://philmaffetone.com/maf-heart-rate-white-paper/

What does this mean for exercise? Technically, by having a higher aerobic base we boost the size and strength of our heart, the concentration of hemoglobin in our blood, the density of our capillaries, and the number of mitochondria in our muscles. The benefits expand beyond the scope of this book but essentially by developing an aerobic base we become healthier inside and out.

What this means for intermittent fasting is that when you are training in a fasted state your body becomes superbly efficient at burning fat for fuel. From an aerobic aspect your body can more efficiently utilize oxygen and this, in turn, makes you more efficient at exercise aerobically or anaerobically. You must first develop your aerobic base to enhance anaerobic exercise. More on this subject goes beyond the scope of this book, but you can check Phil Maffetone's website for more details.

If you are looking to add muscle, fasting can help by increasing the production of certain hormones in your body. Other than weight training and getting the proper amount of sleep regularly, fasting has proven to be one of the most effective methods of increasing human growth hormone, or "HGH". Studies have also suggested that fasting in combination with regular exercise can increase the levels of testosterone in men and women, which is another hormone that can decrease body fat and increase muscle mass. Here are my recommendations for adding muscle:

- Don't push yourself too hard. If you are doing "cardio" exercise, as a test, make sure you are able to carry on a conversation at the same time; otherwise, you may be pushing yourself too hard. When you are doing the exercise slowly but for a long time, that's when your body is becoming more "fat adapted". That's when it is going into a *ketogenic* state. Listen always to your body, and stop if you start to feel dizzy or lightheaded.

- The 16/8 method in particular recommends scheduling your meals for when you plan to finish doing any moderate-to intense exercise. Plan your high intensity workouts for around a time when you are getting ready to break your fast, so you can eat soon thereafter. Properly scheduled, if your workout is very intense, you can follow it with a carbohydrate rich snack.

- If you are lifting weights, make sure you are getting adequate protein or supplementing with adequate BCAAs. "Feast" on meals that are high in protein. Eating protein on a regular basis is vital to muscle growth.

- When planning your meals with workouts in mind, try combining fast-acting simple carbohydrates with a protein that will serve to stabilize your blood sugar after your workout. A banana and some peanut butter is a good example.

Here are some sample routines for nourishment while exercising when using intermittent fasting:

Early Morning Exercise:

- Exercise fasted in the early morning: aerobic or anaerobic. Examples: running or weights

- Take BCAAs afterwards - up to 30 grams before lunch.

- Around Noon: Eat lunch. Aim for about 20-25% of your daily calorie intake.

- Around 3 PM: Snack on high-fat foods, nuts, and seeds.

- Between 4-5 PM: Eat dinner. This should be your largest meal of the day.

- Fast from 8pm until 12 noon the next day.

Lunch Time Exercise:

- Just before Noon: Take up to 30 grams of BCAAs.

- Exercise fasted at lunch: aerobic or anaerobic. Again as examples: running, or weights

- After exercising around 1-2pm: Eat lunch. Aim for 20-25% of your daily calorie intake.

- Around 3-4 PM: Snack on high-fat foods, nuts, and seeds

- Around 6 PM: Eat dinner. This meal's calories should approximate your lunch's.

- Around 8-9 PM: Eat something light. Snack if needed.

- Fast from 9pm or 10pm until 1-2pm the next day.

You will likely not be working out every single day. So, on rest days, your biggest meal of the day should be your first one instead of your last. On rest days, aim for consuming roughly 35-40% of your calories in your first meal, and eat a lot of protein and fat as part of this meal.

My Recommended Supplements

Many trainers recommend taking daily supplements when working out while using intermittent fasting. Our current lifestyle and environment make it challenging if not impossible to ingest all the optimum nutrients via our meals. I recommend some basic supplementation to complete what is missing for the majority of people: Keep it simple - a protein source, an animal source of omega 3 fats, Vitamin D, and a Probiotic. This is the primary approach to fulfilling your body's nutrient requirements, with other supplements filling in the gaps in special circumstances.

- Probiotics: In Paleolithic era, people ate dirt with each meal along with their food intake, including billions of organisms that "came along for the ride." These organisms entered their mouths daily and populated their guts, most being "friendly" bacteria that actually helped digest food and strengthened their immune systems. The problem today is that we don't eat any dirt; we wash everything. Of course, given what today tends to be in and on the dirt around us, it's probably best that we do wash it all away. But in the process we never get a chance to ingest those healthy bacteria that would be helpful for our digestion. I recommend a broad-spectrum probiotic of 20-40 colony forming units (CFU) day. This is the product that I use, Go here to order http://eostre.us/probiotics.

- <u>Fish Oils or Omega-3 Fatty Acids</u>: In primitive times, people obtained the essential fatty acids, both Omega 3 and 6, from dietary sources like wild game, seafood, and from less appetizing sources like grubs and insects. Our modern grain-fed food supply, complete with refined vegetable oils too rich in omega 6, has completely altered the critical balance of Omega3 to Omega6 in our modern diet. Supplementing your diet with pure, pharmaceutical-grade fish oils has proven the best way to re-balance this all-important ratio. The current recommended ratio for Omega6 to Omega3 is 2.4:1. I recommend 800-1,000mg total of EPA/DHA Omega3 per day. Check the labels to make sure the Omega3 you are buying have adequate levels of EPA and DHA. Capsules will work, as long as you don't mind the inconvenience of choking down a big handful of capsules (At most 3 capsules, each dose.) Also if the capsules are way too smelly for you, the solution is to put them in the freezer. This preserves the omega3 longer and also gets rid of the fishy smell. Here is a link to the product that I use, Go here to order http://eostre.us/omega3.

- <u>Vitamin D</u>: Getting adequate vitamin D is essential for your health. With over 3000 binding sites for Vitamin D in every cell of the human body, we are clearly designed to spend time in the sun supplying our body with the rays that aid in the production of this vital pro-hormone. Unfortunately, our modern lifestyles rarely allow for such regular sun exposure, especially in northern climates. <u>Children under the age of one</u> can begin with 5000 IU (International Units), with a dose of 25 IU per lb. of their body weight until reaching the adult dosage. Some people may need more at certain times in their life. Typically, 5000-6000 IU/day will maintain your level of this vitamin in an adequate range for normal physiological function. This is the product that I use: Go here to order http://eostre.us/vitamind

Supplements for Working-Out While Fasting

Let's consider some of the other supplements you may want to add to your workout during fasting. I find they work wonderfully to complement intermittent fasting taken in your eating time frames and along with exercise routine.

Pre-Workout

- Green Tea Extract or ECGC: ECGC stands for *epigallocatechin-3-gallate*. This chemical compound is commonly obtained by drinking Green Tea- from the least processed leaves of the Tea tree. Green tea (straight, unsweetened, without milk) is my favorite drink in the morning pre-workout or pre-work. Lipolysis is the breakdown of stored fat. So, since your goal is to increase fat loss, you will want to increase lipolysis. ECGC is the chemical compound in extract form, and has been shown to block storage of carbohydrates in fat cells, and also aid fat cell apoptosis (fat-cell death). The dose of ECGC should be roughly 325 mg per day to increase the rate of lipolysis. ECGC is a flavonoid, abundant more in green tea, than in black tea, etc. Look for the decaffeinated version. This is the product that I use, Go here to order http://eostre.us/ecgc

- Alpha Lipoic Acid or ALA/lipoic acid: ALA is a strong anti-oxidant which helps protect the cells in our body from breakdown. The benefit of supplementing for fat loss with ALA is its effect on insulin resistance– it lowers it. Just like fasting helps us regulate our insulin better ALA helps make our body less likely to store extra calories as fat. It works by helping us put more calories from the food we eat into muscle instead of fat cells. If I know I'm going to have a big meal or a holiday binge I will reach for more ALA. The dose of ALA should be about 300 mg a day. This is the product that I use, Go here to order http://eostre.us/ALA.

- Caffeine: This may seem odd, but not only can caffeine give you a little boost to get you motivated, but a daily dose of 1 to 3 milligrams per pound of body weight has been shown to increase upper-body strength. Combine it with ECGC to really increase lipolysis even more. Warning: if you are already drinking standard tea or coffee in the morning, you won't need to supplement more caffeine. For many people caffeine does not sit well in their stomach; so try it out first in a small dose.

- Beta-Alanine: This works by decreasing the fatigue associated with buildup of metabolites such as hydrogen ions. What that means for anaerobic exercise is that it can increase anaerobic output without increasing body weight. Want to do heavy weight during your fasted state? Try this! Beta-Alanine increases the amount of *carnosine* stored in the body. Carnosine is an intracellular buffer, which reduces the acidity in the blood, allowing for an increase in exercise performance. Try a dose of 3.2 g to 6.4 g per day. It is best to split the dosage between 2 to 3 smaller servings in a day. This is the product that I use, Go here to order **http://eostre.us/ betaalanine**.

Post-Workout

- Creatine: During intense exercise, creatine is broken down to a *phosphocreatine* releasing *phosphate*, which couples with ADP (*adenosine diphosphate*) to make ATP (*adenosine triphosphate*), which in turn transforms into energy for our body. Supplementing with creatine can not only lead to a boost in energy (both aerobically and anaerobically) but also increases lean muscle mass. A dose of 3 to 5 g per day can lead to a significant increase in strength and power output. (For the vegan athlete: Creatine is found in animal proteins only, but if you body is deficient in this way, taking creatine could really boost performance.) You can try it before or after your workout, but research currently points to it being better as a post-workout supplementation. I recommend a rapid loading phase of creatine followed by a maintenance dose. As a general rule during the loading phase 350 mg(0.35g) per kilogram of body weight (160 mg or 0.16g per pound of body weight) an adult would take about 20 grams of creatine throughout the day mixed with water for the first week and then a maintenance dose of 3 to 5 grams after that. This is the product that I use, Go here to order http://eostre.us/creatine.

- Glutamine: When you start increasing the duration, frequency, and intensity of your workouts, your serum's *glutamine* levels will be affected. This can lead to a decrease in your immune and gut function. Glutamine helps not only to protect your immune system but also prevents a leaky gut. Our gut absorbs glutamine directly producing mucous and *Secretory Imunoglobulin A (SIgA)* which stops undigested foods and toxins from crossing our gut barrier into our bloodstream. Taking 10 g of L-glutamine split into two 5 g doses a day has been found to have a significant impact on the prevention of sickness in general. Take one dose immediately after your workout and the second dose roughly two hours later. You can take powder or capsules depending on your taste buds. This is the product that I use, Go here to order http://eostre.us/glutaminepowder.

Chapter 6: Intermittent Fasting and the Ketogenic Diet

Why is eating fat so good for losing weight? Fats, carbs, and proteins are known as the "macronutrients" and they affect our bodies in different ways. Fat, by far is the most filling and calorie rich food and helps us consume overall less daily by inhibiting the eating of other types of food. In fact, scientifically, 1 gram of protein or carbohydrates provides 4 calories, while 1 gram of fat provides 9 calories.

A ketogenic diet is a high-fat, low-carb method of eating. (It is similar to the Atkins and low-carb diet, but critically different in this way.) Basically, by drastically reducing your body's intake of carbohydrates and replacing them with fat, you are putting your body in a state known as *"ketosis."* Although there are several variations of this diet, normally it consists of eating: 75% fat, 20% protein, and only 5% carbohydrates. I will call these proportions the "standard" ketogenic diet.

There are three other types of well-known ketogenic diets:

1. The *cyclical ketogenic diet* involves having 5 ketogenic days on followed by 2 high-carb days.

2. The *targeted ketogenic diet* (to be described here) is an adaptation that allows you to add carbs around your workouts.

3. Finally, the *high-protein ketogenic diet* is similar to the standard ketogenic diet but includes a lot more protein. For this one, the proportions of the major components is 60% fat, 35% protein, and 5% carbs.

The ketogenic diet and the advent of intermittent fasting were first written about in ancient Greek and Indian medical texts. Hippocrates famous quote: "Let food be thy medicine; and medicine be thy food." was an early indication of the recognition of the importance of diet and nutrition on human overall health. The first study on ketogenic diets was done in France in 1911 on epileptics. At that time epileptic patients were customarily given dangerous doses of *potassium bromide*, which resulted in major toxicity in the brain. They took 20 patients and gave them a low carbohydrate, vegan diet and found that although only a few patients reduced their seizures, the majority of them had improved mental abilities. With the rise of allopathic medicine leading to the discovery of anticonvulsant drugs these nutritional therapies were abandoned. But after seeing 20-30% of adult patients who were epileptic since childhood still with seizures in spite of the medication, the ketogenic diet was reintroduced, again with success. There is now no question the benefit of a ketogenic diet for childhood epileptic syndromes (such as West, Lennox-Gastaut, and Dravet types) has been 30-40% effective based on current medical statistics.

Ketogenic diets have also been shown to help with Parkinson's disease, Alzheimer's disease, and dementia. Currently researches are looking at "ketone bodies" in the human blood and their health benefits. What they have found is *beta-hydroxybutyrate (BHB)*, the most prominent ketone body, has the capacity to cross the blood-brain barrier and to be used for fuel for the brain similar to glucose or sugar. In fact the researchers had shown *BHB* to be <u>more</u> efficient (producing more energy per gram) than glucose. One medical doctor, Mary Newport, made the claim that she has reversed her husband's Alzheimer's disease using coconut oil. One of the main components of a ketogenic diet is consuming large amounts of fat, the most recommended fat being coconut oil. Large research studies are underway at major universities on the effects of coconut oil and *mild chain triglycerides* (a component of coconut oil) on cognitive function and impairment disorders. The results are been very promising.

What does this mean for intermittent fasting, ketogenic diets, weight loss, and performance? It means that if you follow these protocols not only do you improve your physical health but also your mental and emotional health. Hundreds and thousands of people have found relief and healing from many horrible illnesses and conditions by changing what, why, how, and at what frequency they eat.

In general, a ketogenic diet prescribes:

- <u>Avoid these foods</u>: potatoes, rice, breads, pastas, cereals, grains, tortillas (flour or corn), fruit and fruit juices, soy products, fried foods, processed foods, refined sugars ("sodas"), chips and cookies, crackers and dips, alcohol, artificial ingredients, and artificial sweeteners. I know this sounds like a lot but stay with me.

- <u>Stick to these foods</u>: Meats, fish, eggs, butter, nuts and seeds, coconut and avocado, cheese, heavy and sour cream, chicken and beef bone broths, low-carb veggies such as cauliflower, celery, onion, cabbage, bell peppers, squash, spinach, zucchini, and water, coffee or tea. Try to stick to organic, grass-fed, and cage-free products if possible. It is best to stick to whole, single-ingredient foods for your meals. For instance, dark chocolate (~70% cacao) is a good treat for people seeking to go into ketosis. Use this lists as a guide. There is "a ton" of information on ketonic diets out there on the Internet, including many excellent ketonic recipes.

Similarly to intermittent fasting, a ketogenic diet has been shown to increase insulin sensitivity in the cells of the body, which lowers blood sugar. An advantage over traditional diets is its emphasis on the assimilation of fats of various types. Since intermittent fasting and the ketogenic diet have similar impacts on your body (getting it to use stored fat as energy instead of the food you just consumed) it only makes sense to try combining them.

If you are interested in trying intermittent fasting while using the ketogenic diet, keep the following things in mind:

- Do not start both of them at the same time. Learn from the mistakes of others, and from mine. Your body needs to get adapted to the ketogenic diet before it is required to go through longer periods of time without eating. I recommend at first taking two weeks to get accustomed to the ketogenic diet without doing any purposeful fasting, and subsequently combine it with an intermittent fasting schedule best suited for you.

- Start out slow, and go with what feels naturally. You might automatically begin to detoxify or cleanse out in what is called a "Herxheimer reaction". Once your body adjusts to using up fat reserves and becomes "fat-adapted" you will start to feel less hungry. Try starting out by not snacking between meals before moving on to skipping a whole meal.

- <u>Keep yourself busy</u>. Do not spend a lot of time hanging in and around your kitchen or supermarkets, and plan plenty of things to do to keep yourself busy. Do not surround yourself with temptations and get "out of the house" as often as you can.

- <u>Cook and prepare several of your meals in advance</u>. It's always easier to sit down and eat when you have prepared efficiently. Food preparation is much easier if you eat the same things 3 to 4 times a week. Getting a crock-pot was one of the best investments I ever made. Without much time involved, it helps me to cook lots of food, and I store it for a later time. One of my favorite cookware inventions of late is the Instapot. Go here to orderhttp://amzn.to/2fpf3j2

- <u>Do not expect your new diet and intermittent fasting to fix everything</u> you might be ailing from. It definitely will help you lose weight and to be healthier. But, simultaneously, you should also be working on your stress levels and on getting enough sleep (you would know when you need more sleep, and it varies from person to person.) And it's best if you can include purposeful exercise in your weekly schedule.

In summary, when you are doing a ketogenic diet, remember that when it is time to eat, you need meals that are high in healthy fats and low in carbohydrates.

Here is one of my favorite recipes for a great "ketogenic" snack. I like to pick cooking something flavorful, easy to make, and quick, just like in this recipe below:

Chocolate and Peanut Butter Fat Bombs - Delicious!

What you'll need:

1. A fuel source and container (pot and stove)
2. Coconut Oil (Dr. Bronner's is the best tasting Go here to order http://eostre.us/bronnerscoconut)
3. Raw Cacao Powder (Go here to order http://eostre.us/cacao)
4. Organic Peanut Butter (Go here to order http://eostre.us/peanutbutter)
5. Stevia Liquid (Go here to order http://eostre.us/stevia)
6. Non-stick cupcake tray (Go here to order http://eostre.us/nonsticktray)

Ingredients:

1. 1 cup organic virgin coconut oil
2. 1 cup organic peanut butter, or almond butter
3. 4 Tablespoons (1/4 cup) raw cacao powder
4. 2 to 3 drops of Stevia, or Cinnamon liquid

Instructions:

1. Melt the coconut in a pot over low heat
2. Add the peanut butter and cacao
3. Add the Stevia or cinnamon
4. Wait for everything to melt. Avoid boiling

5. Pour into a glass or preferably a Pyrex measuring cup

6. Pour into a cupcake tray, and place in the freezer

7. Allow them to cool for 1 hour or so, and... enjoy!

Chapter 7: Incorrect Myths About Intermittent Fasting

There may be many reasons why you might hesitate in starting an intermittent fast, but many of them may be based on inaccurate ideas about eating and fasting that are often circulated in society, television shows, etc. Also, some corporations marketing supplements, or "fitness" products, or highly processed foods, spend millions of dollars to try to convince people that they need their products in order to be healthy and happy. Let's go ahead and debunk some of these common falsehoods turned into myths by constant repetition.

Skipping Breakfast is Bad for You and Will Make You "Fat" (Obese)

According to this mindset, not only is skipping breakfast terrible, but it will also make you fat! It is true that people who skip breakfast are more likely to be overweight, but that is due to their other lifestyle choices, not to regularly skipping breakfast. Breakfast-skippers are statistically likely to be on some idealistic diet which they do not follow consistently. And they statistically also have less concern for their overall health. For them, the imposed idea of being on a diet often results in binge eating later. If you are skipping breakfast as part of a controlled and intentional intermittent fasting there is no reason that would make you fat. In fact, current research has shown that before your breakfast in the morning your insulin levels which normally control your blood sugar, are low. When your insulin is low you also

47

produce more *Human Growth Hormone (HGH)* which helps burn fat, build muscle, and slow the aging process. So skipping breakfast, by itself does not make you gradually "fat" or "obese".

You Will Feel Too Hungry

No one wants to walk around feeling hungry all day. It's true that in the beginning you are going to feel really hungry, but the feeling is not going to last. Why? Almost everything that makes up our lives is based on the habits we have formed. Habits replace the use of willpower in order to accomplish something we want. Many of the times your body signals to you that you are hungry it is really just reacting to a habit you have developed of eating at a particular time. It may be difficult to ignore these hunger triggers initially. But keep in mind that it can take 30 to 60 days for a new habit to form and replace the old one. Hang in there and it will be worth it. Feelings of hunger are often just cravings for either sugars or carbohydrates (which the body turns into sugars). Give your body time to draw energy from other sources and the feelings of hunger during fasting periods should normally go away.

You Will Develop Deficiencies

When you are fasting, you are simply teaching your body to expect nutrients during certain parts of the day. You will not be missing out on essential vitamins or minerals. The ketogenic diet provides adequate nutrition for your body. If this is a major concern for you, look into taking a multivitamin on your fasting days. It is not be considered a reason to avoid trying an intermittent fast.

Only Muscle Will Be Lost

The reason our bodies store fat is to use it as an energy source when lots of energy is needed later. Remember our hunter-gatherer ancestors who had to hunt and therefore walk or run far to find game. If they could do it, so can we. Fat is a high-energy molecule. Remember that 1 gram contains more than two times the energy of a carbohydrate or protein gram. It only makes sense for your body to preferentially burn stored fat when it needs more energy than you are eating at the moment. About 85% of our body's calorie reserves are in fat stores, and 14% are in the form of protein, to maintain our muscle mass. That is why you must continue to intake adequate amounts of protein or protein components - amino acids (called BCAAs in tablet form) - which your body combines to form many kinds of proteins it needs. Taking BCAAs is an alternative and very practical way to continue to get the protein you need to maintain and build muscle mass.

Your Blood Sugar Will Get Out of Control

The simple fact is: if you are healthy, your blood sugar levels are well regulated and maintained. Obviously this applies to people who are not diabetic or dealing with other illnesses. Normally, blood sugar level will not go up or down significantly if you go without food for a 16-hour stretch or even a whole day. But your insulin levels may fluctuate, and that's why our goal is to eventually reduce "insulin resistance" caused by too much intake of sugars and carbs. Overcoming insulin resistance (the body state in which the body cells begin to resist taking-in any more sugar) is the key to becoming "fat adapted". Your body will have so much more energy to heal, repair, and metabolize efficiently and effectively. Again, our ancestors sometimes had to go long stretches when they did not have food readily available, so they had to push themselves further than what mere carbohydrate energy could provide, and for them it was considered normal (and it is) for their bodies to run on fat and handle great energy bursts.

Fasting Will Ruin Your Aerobic Training Performance

Research on people fasting during Ramadan, a Muslim holy month that requires fasting during the day and allows eating only at night, showed that it had an insignificant effect on their performance during aerobic activities. Nevertheless, during Ramadan, fluids are also restricted. If you are simply intermittent fasting and keep yourself hydrated during intermittent fasting, the lack of food intake should not impact your exercise training performance one single bit.

Fasting Will Ruin Your Weight Training Performance

Again this is not true. With a natural boost in human growth hormone (HGH) in the morning and an adequate supply of protein via BCAAs throughout the morning, you should be fine. If you need more energy to get through a workout drink tea or coffee without sugars.

Your Cholesterol Will Increase if You Eat High-Fat

"Ok, so whether I have high cholesterol or not, eating a diet of 75% of fat should be bad news, right?" Not necessarily. New research is out regarding LDL- called the "bad cholesterol", as opposed to HDL- called the "good cholesterol".

Recent research has shown that LDL can be measured in two ways: One, called LDL-C, measures the concentration of cholesterol carried in a person's blood at that moment. And the second test (called LDL-P) measures the number (and size) LDL particles in the blood. But what is of greatest interest is the size of the LDL particles. Current research has shown that the LDL particle size is a far more precise indicator for the potential of cardiovascular disease (CVD) than total LDL cholesterol particle count. The smaller the LDL particle size on the LDL-P test, the greater the health risk. The larger the LDL particle size on the LDL-P test, the lesser the health risk. Concentration of LDL alone is not as precise an indicator.)

Confused yet? In short, eating more good fat can raise your cholesterol, but it also raises the size of your LDL particles. You might ask: "Is this good for me?" As we stated before: current research is pointing to the benefits of high-fat diets for Alzheimer's, and other neurological disorders. Our brain is 60% fat by weight. So, facetiously speaking, could it be that the more fat we eat, the smarter we could get?

Chapter 8: If Intermittent Fasting Isn't Working For You

There are certain groups of people who in their current condition should not attempt intermittent fasting, or any fasting for that matter. The incorrect myths previously discussed could have arisen from observed effects on the following categories or health conditions of some people, who should not have been fasting in the first place, considering their particular, special, condition:

- <u>Pregnant or Nursing Women</u>: Babies need a constant and intense flow of nutrients, and by fasting a pregnant or nursing woman may affect the growth of her baby in a negative way.

- <u>Diabetic or Hypoglycemic People</u>: If you suffer from one of these conditions it may still be possible to try intermittent fasting but only under close supervision of a doctor. These people need to get the proper nutrients at the proper time, so their bodies may initially not be compatible with any kind of fasting program.

- <u>People with Chronic Illnesses, or Recovering</u>: If your body is dealing with above-normal duress more than the average person, intermittent fasting may slow down your healing, or even cause some damage. Consulting a physician is recommended if you are not sure whether you are healthy enough to begin an intermittent fasting regime.

- <u>People with Eating Disorders</u>: Sufferers of *anorexia nervosa* and *bulimia nervosa* should not try to restrict their food intake during any intervals of time due to the possible negative impact(s) on their mental health.

- <u>People with Chronic Stress or Sleep Disorders</u>: Take care of the stress or sleep deprivation first, or else the stress of fasting may end up being too much for your body.

- <u>Children</u>: When children are in a growth stage, their bodies require much nourishment. Never have a child or teenager under the age of 18 try intermittent fasting.

If you are not in any of the previously mentioned categories and intermittent fasting has not given you results, that could be due to some of the following possibilities:

- <u>You may be eating too much during your permitted time-windows</u>. It's important to look at not only how much you are eating, but also what you are eating. The ketogenic diet example in this book is a great start. When all is said, for most everyone, losing weight is astonishingly simple: You just have to burn more calories than you consume.

- <u>You are expecting too much too soon in the process</u>. The bathroom scale is not the best tool to measure your results. The number on the scale could very well not be going down because you are gaining muscle, or because you are carrying some extra water weight, or because you obviously just ate a meal, etc. Try to weigh yourself regularly once a week but do it at the same time of day each instance. Also invest in a bioimpedence device that measures just body fat percentage. What is relevant for you is the loss in body fat percentage, rather than overall weight loss. For the product I use: Go here to order http://eostre.us/bodyfat

- <u>Your diet might be really unhealthy</u>. If you are eating highly processed foods during your eating periods, that may prevent you from losing weight. It may also have negative impacts on your health. Look into a ketogenic diet as described in this book (or the Paleo Diet), and you should start seeing results, assuming dieting is for you.

- <u>You're not clear on your motivation</u>. If you are submitting to temptation too easily, cheat in your fasting regime frequently, or are not sticking to your adopted intermittent fasting schedule, try making a list of the reasons you wanted to start it in the first place. Creating a journal is a great first step to seeing any progress both inside and outside the body. Refer to it when you are considering "throwing in the towel". It will also help you to be prepared to answer the pessimistic or negative people in your life who may not understand why you are doing what you are doing.

- <u>You tried to do too much, too fast</u>. If you tried to completely change your life overnight, you are going to set yourself up for failure. Do not overtax your willpower. Implement in stages your new plan for living. You will be healthier in the end if you start out slowly and be able to stick with it, rather than if you subjected yourself to the max for two weeks and then just quit.

Conclusion

Thanks again for taking the time to download this book!

You should now have a good understanding of several methods for intermittent fasting, a good start on ketogenic diets, and know how to implement these methods into your lifestyle, whether you exercise much or not. By following the advice and tips in this book you should be able to reap all of the exciting benefits intermittent fasting has to offer. After starting your intermittent fasting for a few cycles, you will find it hard later to imagine going back to life without it.

Going on a fasting program means making a definite change in your life. What's important is that you must embrace that change to make it become a lifestyle choice for you. The change has to come <u>from you</u>, and won't come <u>to you</u>. That is, from <u>within</u> you, not from <u>outside</u> you. Food choice is one of the hardest things to change in our lives but also one of the most rewarding things we can do to change our health and vitality.

Yours in health, Dr. Foss

www.fatadapteddoc.com, www.puravidasanantonio.com,

Thank You

Reader, maybe you picked up multiple books on the topic of intermittent fasting and gave mine a shot. One of the greatest gifts one can give is the gift of knowledge, and sharing this knowledge was my ultimate goal in creating this book.

If you enjoyed this book, please take the time to leave me a good review on Amazon. I would appreciate your honest feedback, whatever it is. It would encourage me and help me continue producing high-quality books that people might use to live content or happier lives. So if you enjoyed it, please let me know!

Simply leave a review here, https://www.amazon.com/dp/B01LRHZ70M, or check out my website: www.fatadapteddoc.com for free glimpses of my other authored books to date.